Healing with Herb

Healing with Herb

Matthew Petchinsky

Healing with Herb: Cannabis and Hydrocephalus
By: Matthew Petchinsky

Introduction

Hydrocephalus, often referred to as *"water on the brain,"* is a complex and potentially life-altering neurological condition that affects individuals of all ages—from newborn infants to the elderly. It is characterized by an abnormal accumulation of cerebrospinal fluid (CSF) within the brain's interconnected cavities known as ventricles. Under normal conditions, CSF flows freely through these spaces, cushioning the brain, delivering nutrients, and removing waste. However, when this delicate system is disrupted—either due to overproduction, impaired absorption, or blockage of flow—fluid begins to accumulate. This buildup increases intracranial pressure, which can lead to brain tissue damage, severe neurological symptoms, and, if untreated, life-threatening complications.

Over the decades, medical science has developed effective interventions for managing hydrocephalus, with surgical techniques such as shunt implantation and endoscopic third ventriculostomy (ETV) revolutionizing patient care. These procedures have saved countless lives, enabling many to live long and productive years despite the diagnosis. Yet, these solutions are not without their challenges. Shunts, while life-saving, are prone to infection, mechanical failure, and the need for repeated revisions over a patient's lifetime. ETV procedures, though less invasive, are not suitable for every case and can also require follow-up interventions. In addition, the ongoing management of hydrocephalus often involves navigating chronic pain, inflammation, emotional strain, and other secondary symptoms that can significantly affect quality of life.

It is within this context that alternative and complementary therapies have begun to capture interest—particularly cannabis-based medicine. Once surrounded by legal barriers and social stigma, cannabis is now being re-evaluated through the lens of modern science. Research is increasingly highlighting its potential therapeutic properties, particularly for conditions involving chronic pain, inflammation, neurodegeneration, and sleep disturbances—all of which are relevant to the lived experience of many hydrocephalus patients.

Cannabis contains a variety of active compounds known as cannabinoids, with tetrahydrocannabinol (THC) and cannabidiol (CBD) being the most widely studied. These compounds interact with the body's endocannabinoid system—a network of receptors and signaling molecules that helps regulate pain, mood, immune response, and neurological function. Through this interaction, cannabis has shown promise in alleviating persistent headaches, reducing inflammation, protecting neural tissue from damage, improving sleep, and easing anxiety—symptoms and challenges that frequently accompany hydrocephalus.

The purpose of this book is not to promote cannabis as a cure for hydrocephalus, but rather to explore its potential role as a complementary therapy alongside established medical treatments. Drawing upon existing research, patient experiences, and medical perspectives, we will examine how cannabis might fit into a holistic care plan for hydrocephalus patients.

Whether you are a patient seeking symptom relief, a caregiver searching for additional support strategies, or a healthcare professional looking to expand your understanding of cannabis in neurological care, this book offers a balanced, evidence-based, and practical guide. Together, we will navigate the science, the potential benefits, the limitations, and the responsible approaches to integrating cannabis into hydrocephalus management—always with the goal of improving quality of life and empowering informed decision-making.

Chapter 1 – Understanding Hydrocephalus

Hydrocephalus, while commonly summarized as *"water on the brain,"* is far more complex than its nickname suggests. It is a neurological condition in which cerebrospinal fluid (CSF)—a clear, nutrient-rich fluid that surrounds and cushions the brain and spinal cord—accumulates abnormally in the brain's ventricular system. This excess fluid increases intracranial pressure, which can damage delicate brain tissue and disrupt normal brain function.

The impact of hydrocephalus varies dramatically between individuals, depending on factors such as age at onset, type of hydrocephalus, cause, severity, and the speed at which fluid builds up. Some individuals may require emergency medical intervention within hours of symptom onset, while others may develop symptoms more gradually over months or years.

The Role of Cerebrospinal Fluid

To understand hydrocephalus, it is essential to appreciate the role of CSF. This fluid is continuously produced within the ventricles, circulates through the brain and spinal cord, and is eventually absorbed into the bloodstream. CSF serves several critical functions:

- **Protection:** Acts as a shock absorber, safeguarding the brain and spinal cord from injury.
- **Nutrient Delivery:** Transports vital nutrients to brain cells.
- **Waste Removal:** Removes metabolic waste products from the brain's environment.
- **Pressure Regulation:** Helps maintain stable pressure within the skull.

In a healthy system, the production, circulation, and absorption of CSF are in balance. Hydrocephalus occurs when this balance is disrupted—either due to overproduction, blocked circulation pathways, or reduced absorption.

Types of Hydrocephalus

Hydrocephalus is not a single condition but a group of related disorders, classified based on their cause and how CSF flow is disrupted.

1. **Congenital Hydrocephalus**
   - Present at birth.
   - Often caused by abnormal brain development or genetic conditions.
   - Can also be linked to prenatal infections or other environmental factors during pregnancy.
   - Frequently detected due to rapid head growth in infants.
2. **Acquired Hydrocephalus**
   - Develops after birth as a result of injury, tumor, infection (e.g., meningitis), or bleeding in the brain.
   - Can occur at any age.
3. **Communicating Hydrocephalus**
   - CSF can still flow between the ventricles, but its absorption into the bloodstream is impaired.
   - Often associated with meningitis, hemorrhage, or post-surgical complications.
4. **Non-Communicating (Obstructive) Hydrocephalus**
   - Caused by a blockage in the ventricular system that prevents CSF from flowing freely.
   - Frequently linked to structural abnormalities or tumors.
5. **Normal Pressure Hydrocephalus (NPH)**
   - Primarily affects older adults.
   - Despite the name, CSF pressure is not always within normal range; the defining feature is gradual symptom progression.
   - Classic triad of symptoms: difficulty walking, urinary incontinence, and cognitive decline.

Symptoms by Age Group

Infants

- Rapid increase in head size.
- Bulging soft spot (fontanel) on the head.
- Vomiting, irritability, sleepiness.
- Seizures in some cases.

Children & Adolescents

- Chronic headaches, often worse in the morning.
- Double vision or difficulty focusing.
- Decline in academic performance due to cognitive changes.
- Problems with balance and coordination.

Adults

- Persistent headaches and nausea.
- Difficulty concentrating and memory impairment.
- Loss of bladder control.
- Personality or mood changes.

Older Adults (NPH)

- Shuffling gait or difficulty walking.
- Urinary urgency or incontinence.
- Slowed thinking, confusion, or dementia-like symptoms.

Causes and Risk Factors

While hydrocephalus can occur without an identifiable cause, several factors increase the risk:

- Brain or spinal cord tumors.
- Infections affecting the central nervous system.
- Brain hemorrhage, especially in premature infants.
- Severe head injury.
- Genetic predispositions affecting brain development.

Diagnosis

Timely diagnosis is critical. The process typically involves:

- **Neurological Examination:** To assess symptoms and identify potential deficits in vision, coordination, memory, or movement.
- **Imaging Studies:** MRI and CT scans are the gold standards for visualizing CSF buildup, identifying blockages, and assessing brain structure.
- **Intracranial Pressure Monitoring:** In select cases, pressure inside the skull may be measured directly.
- **Specialized Testing for NPH:** May include lumbar puncture (spinal tap) to remove CSF and observe symptom improvement.

The Importance of Understanding Hydrocephalus

While the condition itself may be lifelong, early intervention and careful management can dramatically improve quality of life. Understanding hydrocephalus in detail enables patients, families, and care providers to:

- Recognize symptoms early.
- Make informed treatment decisions.
- Plan for both immediate and long-term care.

This foundational knowledge is essential as we explore in later chapters how cannabis—when used responsibly and under medical supervision—might complement traditional therapies, address difficult-to-manage symptoms, and improve overall well-being for individuals living with hydrocephalus.

Chapter 2 – Conventional Treatments and Their Limitations

The management of hydrocephalus has evolved significantly over the past century, moving from high-risk and often ineffective procedures to refined surgical techniques that can dramatically improve survival and quality of life. While these treatments have saved countless lives, they are not without risks, complications, and long-term maintenance challenges.

This chapter provides an in-depth look at the most common conventional treatments for hydrocephalus, how they work, their advantages, and the limitations that often drive patients and caregivers to explore complementary approaches such as cannabis therapy.

Primary Goals of Conventional Treatment

The central aim in treating hydrocephalus is to restore the balance of cerebrospinal fluid (CSF) within the brain and spinal cord. Specifically, treatment seeks to:

- Relieve intracranial pressure.
- Restore normal CSF circulation.
- Prevent or minimize further brain tissue damage.
- Alleviate symptoms to improve daily functioning and quality of life.

Since hydrocephalus is most often caused by a blockage or absorption problem rather than overproduction of CSF, treatments primarily focus on rerouting or improving fluid drainage rather than reducing CSF production.

Surgical Interventions

1. Shunt Systems

Shunt systems are the most widely used treatment for hydrocephalus. They consist of three main components:

- **Ventricular Catheter:** A thin tube inserted into one of the brain's ventricles to collect excess CSF.
- **Valve Mechanism:** Regulates the flow of CSF, ensuring it drains at the correct rate. Valves may be fixed-pressure or adjustable (programmable).
- **Distal Catheter:** Directs CSF to another part of the body—most commonly the peritoneal cavity in the abdomen—where it can be reabsorbed.

Common Shunt Types:

- **Ventriculoperitoneal (VP) Shunt:** CSF drains into the abdominal cavity.
- **Ventriculoatrial (VA) Shunt:** CSF drains into the right atrium of the heart.
- **Ventriculopleural Shunt:** CSF drains into the pleural cavity around the lungs.
- **Lumboperitoneal (LP) Shunt:** CSF is drained from the lumbar spinal canal to the abdomen, often used when ventricles are not enlarged.

Advantages:

- Effective for both acute and chronic hydrocephalus.
- Adjustable shunts allow for non-invasive pressure setting changes.

Limitations and Risks:

- **Infection:** Shunt infections can be life-threatening and require immediate treatment.
- **Blockage:** Debris or tissue growth can clog the shunt, causing recurrence of symptoms.
- **Over- or Under-Drainage:** Can lead to headaches, subdural hematomas, or ventricular collapse.
- **Frequent Revisions:** Many patients, especially children, require multiple surgeries over their lifetime.

2. Endoscopic Third Ventriculostomy (ETV)

ETV is a minimally invasive procedure that creates a small opening in the floor of the third ventricle, allowing CSF to bypass an obstruction and flow toward absorption pathways at the brain's surface.

Best Suited For:

- Non-communicating (obstructive) hydrocephalus.
- Patients with aqueductal stenosis or certain tumor-related blockages.

Advantages:

- No implanted device, reducing infection and mechanical failure risks.
- Often effective long-term if the stoma (opening) remains open.

Limitations and Risks:

- Not suitable for all types of hydrocephalus, especially those involving absorption issues.
- Stoma can close over time, requiring repeat surgery.
- Risk of injury to surrounding brain structures during the procedure.

Non-Surgical Medical Management

1. Medications

While not a definitive solution, certain medications can temporarily reduce CSF production or manage symptoms:

- **Diuretics** (e.g., acetazolamide, furosemide): Reduce CSF production by inhibiting carbonic anhydrase.
- **Corticosteroids:** Used in cases involving inflammation-related swelling.

Limitations:

- Often a temporary measure before surgery.
- Side effects may include electrolyte imbalance, fatigue, or gastrointestinal issues.
- Not suitable for long-term management in most cases.

Challenges and Limitations of Conventional Treatments

1. Lifelong Dependence on Medical Devices

Patients with shunts often remain dependent on them for life, facing the constant possibility of malfunction or infection.

2. Quality-of-Life Concerns

Even when hydrocephalus is "managed" surgically, patients may still experience chronic headaches, fatigue, cognitive changes, or emotional distress.

3. Surgical and Post-Surgical Risks

Every surgery carries anesthesia risks, bleeding risks, and the potential for neurological injury.

4. Limited Effectiveness in Certain Cases

For example, in some forms of normal pressure hydrocephalus, symptom improvement after shunting may be partial or temporary.

5. Healthcare Burden

Multiple revisions, hospital stays, and follow-ups can place a significant emotional, financial, and logistical burden on patients and families.

Why Some Patients Look Beyond Conventional Care

The limitations of surgery and the side effects of medications often prompt individuals to explore complementary options. These may include physical therapy, dietary changes, stress-reduction techniques, and—more recently—medical cannabis. The potential for cannabis to address pain, inflammation, and mood disturbances without invasive intervention has sparked growing interest among patients, researchers, and some clinicians.

Chapter 3 – Cannabis: Plant Profile and Medical Potential

Cannabis is one of the most studied and debated medicinal plants in the world today. Known scientifically as *Cannabis sativa L.*, the plant has been cultivated for thousands of years for medicinal, nutritional, and industrial purposes. Its therapeutic potential lies in a unique set of compounds called cannabinoids, which interact with the body's endocannabinoid system—a complex regulatory network that influences pain perception, immune response, mood, and neurological health.

In recent decades, advances in both cannabis research and medical legalization have reignited interest in its role as a therapeutic agent. For individuals with neurological conditions such as hydrocephalus, cannabis presents a compelling area of exploration due to its analgesic, anti-inflammatory, and neuroprotective properties.

Historical Context of Cannabis Use

Ancient Civilizations

- **China (circa 2700 BCE):** Cannabis was recorded in ancient Chinese pharmacopeias as a treatment for pain, inflammation, and various ailments.
- **India:** The Ayurvedic tradition used cannabis for sleep disorders, digestive issues, and as a stress-relieving tonic, often in spiritual and ceremonial contexts.
- **Egypt and the Middle East:** Evidence from ancient scrolls and archaeological finds indicates cannabis was used for treating inflammation and eye conditions.

Spread to the Western World

- During the 19th century, cannabis extracts entered Western medicine, prescribed for migraines, seizures, and muscle spasms.
- By the early 20th century, it was included in the U.S. Pharmacopeia.
- Legal restrictions and prohibition in the mid-1900s halted much of the research, only to be revived in the late 20th century as public attitudes shifted.

The Cannabis Plant: Anatomy and Key Components

Cannabis is a chemically rich plant with hundreds of biologically active compounds. The most important groups include:

1. Cannabinoids

These are plant-derived molecules that mimic the body's naturally occurring endocannabinoids.

- **Tetrahydrocannabinol (THC):** The primary psychoactive cannabinoid. Known for its euphoric effects, but also valued for its pain relief, appetite stimulation, and anti-nausea properties.
- **Cannabidiol (CBD):** Non-psychoactive and widely studied for anti-inflammatory, anti-anxiety, and neuroprotective effects.
- **Minor Cannabinoids:** Compounds such as cannabigerol (CBG), cannabinol (CBN), and tetrahydrocannabivarin (THCV) show promise for niche therapeutic uses, including neuroprotection and appetite regulation.

2. Terpenes

Aromatic compounds that give cannabis its distinctive scent and may influence therapeutic effects through the "entourage effect." Examples:

- **Myrcene:** Sedative, muscle relaxant, analgesic.
- **Limonene:** Uplifting, anti-anxiety, antibacterial.
- **Pinene:** Anti-inflammatory, memory-supporting.

3. Flavonoids

Plant pigments with antioxidant and anti-inflammatory properties. Some cannabis-specific flavonoids, called cannaflavins, may offer anti-inflammatory effects stronger than aspirin in lab studies.

The Endocannabinoid System (ECS): How Cannabis Works in the Body

The ECS is a network of receptors, endogenous cannabinoids, and enzymes that help regulate balance (homeostasis) in the body. It influences:

- Pain perception.
- Inflammation levels.
- Mood and stress response.
- Appetite and digestion.
- Neuroprotection and neural repair.

Main ECS Components:

- **CB1 Receptors:** Found primarily in the brain and central nervous system; regulate pain, memory, and motor control.
- **CB2 Receptors:** Located mainly in the immune system; regulate inflammation and immune responses.
- **Endocannabinoids:** Natural cannabinoids made by the body, such as anandamide (AEA) and 2-AG.
- **Enzymes:** Break down endocannabinoids once they are no longer needed.

Cannabis-derived cannabinoids (THC, CBD, etc.) can bind to or influence these receptors, altering physiological processes in ways that can be therapeutic for certain conditions.

Medical Benefits Relevant to Hydrocephalus

Cannabis's potential therapeutic roles in hydrocephalus care stem from several pharmacological effects:

1. Analgesia (Pain Relief)

- THC's interaction with CB1 receptors modulates pain perception in the brain and spinal cord.
- CBD may reduce pain indirectly by decreasing inflammation and enhancing serotonin receptor activity.

2. Anti-Inflammatory Effects

- CB2 receptor activation can reduce immune-driven inflammation in the brain and other tissues.
- CBD's ability to downregulate pro-inflammatory cytokines may help manage inflammation associated with secondary causes of hydrocephalus.

3. Neuroprotection

- Both THC and CBD show antioxidant properties, reducing oxidative stress that contributes to neuronal damage.
- Cannabinoids may help preserve neural function by supporting cerebral blood flow and reducing excitotoxicity (overstimulation of nerve cells).

4. Adjunctive Symptom Management

- Improving sleep quality in patients with pain or anxiety.
- Supporting appetite in patients whose nutrition is impacted by chronic illness.
- Reducing nausea and vomiting associated with medications or secondary conditions.

Safety and Considerations

While cannabis holds promise, it is not without potential drawbacks:

- **Psychoactive effects** (especially with THC) may not be well-tolerated by all patients.
- **Drug interactions** are possible with medications used to manage hydrocephalus symptoms.
- **Cognitive effects** may be more pronounced in younger patients or with high THC exposure.

Responsible medical use involves starting with low doses, using lab-tested products, and working with healthcare providers experienced in cannabinoid medicine.

Conclusion

Cannabis is a complex plant with a long history of medicinal use and a growing body of modern research supporting its potential in neurological care. For hydrocephalus patients, its pain-relieving, anti-inflammatory, and neuroprotective effects offer a possible complementary approach to conventional treatments.

Chapter 4 – Cannabis and the Human Body

Understanding how cannabis interacts with the human body begins with an appreciation of its primary target: the endocannabinoid system (ECS). This intricate signaling network, discovered in the early 1990s, plays a pivotal role in regulating balance—or *homeostasis*—across multiple physiological systems. It is active in all humans regardless of cannabis use and influences processes ranging from pain perception to immune function, appetite regulation, emotional health, and neural protection.

For individuals living with hydrocephalus, the ECS is of particular interest because many of the challenges associated with the condition—pain, inflammation, and neural stress—are processes modulated by this system. Cannabis-derived compounds, known as phytocannabinoids, can interact with ECS pathways in ways that may help alleviate certain symptoms or improve quality of life.

The Endocannabinoid System: Core Components

The ECS is composed of three main elements:

1. Endocannabinoids

These are naturally occurring molecules produced by the body that resemble the active compounds found in cannabis. The two best-studied endocannabinoids are:

- **Anandamide (AEA):** Often called the "bliss molecule," it plays a role in mood regulation, appetite, memory, and pain modulation.
- **2-Arachidonoylglycerol (2-AG):** More abundant than anandamide, it is involved in immune system regulation and inflammation control.

2. Cannabinoid Receptors

These receptors are embedded in cell membranes throughout the body and serve as docking points for cannabinoids:

- **CB1 Receptors:** Found primarily in the brain and central nervous system. They influence mood, pain perception, appetite, and memory.
- **CB2 Receptors:** Located mostly in immune cells and peripheral tissues. They play a critical role in regulating inflammation and immune responses.

3. Enzymes

Specialized enzymes create and break down endocannabinoids as needed:

- **FAAH (Fatty Acid Amide Hydrolase):** Breaks down anandamide.
- **MAGL (Monoacylglycerol Lipase):** Breaks down 2-AG.

How Cannabis Interacts with the ECS

Cannabis contains over 100 phytocannabinoids that can influence ECS activity. The two most widely studied are tetrahydrocannabinol (THC) and cannabidiol (CBD), but other minor cannabinoids also contribute to therapeutic effects.

THC (Tetrahydrocannabinol)

- **Mechanism:** THC binds directly to CB1 receptors in the brain and CB2 receptors in the immune system.
- **Effects:** Produces psychoactive sensations ("high"), but also relieves pain, stimulates appetite, reduces nausea, and may help with muscle relaxation.
- **Relevance to Hydrocephalus:** By acting on CB1 receptors, THC can modulate pain signals and may reduce the intensity of chronic headaches.

CBD (Cannabidiol)

- **Mechanism:** CBD does not strongly bind to CB1 or CB2 receptors. Instead, it modulates receptor activity indirectly, inhibits FAAH to increase anandamide levels, and interacts with other receptor systems such as serotonin and vanilloid receptors.
- **Effects:** Non-psychoactive, with anti-inflammatory, anxiolytic, and neuroprotective properties.
- **Relevance to Hydrocephalus:** CBD's anti-inflammatory action may help reduce inflammation in the brain or spinal tissues, while its neuroprotective effects could support long-term brain health.

The Entourage Effect

Cannabinoids often work best when combined with other cannabinoids and terpenes found in the plant. This synergistic interaction, called the entourage effect, may enhance therapeutic benefits compared to isolated compounds.

Physiological Effects Relevant to Hydrocephalus

1. Pain Modulation
Both THC and CBD can alter the perception of pain by influencing neural pathways in the brain and spinal cord. For hydrocephalus patients who experience chronic headaches, this modulation can be a significant quality-of-life improvement.

2. Anti-Inflammatory Action
By activating CB2 receptors and influencing immune cell function, cannabinoids can reduce inflammatory processes. In hydrocephalus—especially in cases secondary to infection, trauma, or hemorrhage—this may help minimize tissue damage.

3. Neuroprotection
Cannabinoids act as antioxidants, helping to protect brain cells from oxidative stress and free radical damage. This is particularly important for individuals with hydrocephalus, where elevated intracranial pressure can stress neural tissue over time.

4. Emotional Regulation
Hydrocephalus can bring emotional challenges, including anxiety and depression. CBD's influence on serotonin receptors may help stabilize mood, while THC at low doses may promote relaxation.

5. Sleep Support
Sleep disruption is common in chronic neurological conditions. THC can help reduce the time it takes to fall asleep, while CBD may improve sleep quality by reducing anxiety and pain.

Potential Risks and Side Effects

While cannabis can be beneficial, it is not without risks:

- **Cognitive Impairment:** High THC doses may impair short-term memory and concentration.
- **Psychoactive Reactions:** THC can cause anxiety or paranoia in some individuals, especially at high doses.
- **Drug Interactions:** Cannabinoids can alter the metabolism of certain prescription medications.
- **Tolerance and Dependence:** Frequent use of THC can lead to tolerance, requiring higher doses for the same effect.

Optimizing Cannabis Use for Hydrocephalus Patients

1. Start Low and Go Slow

Begin with a low dose and increase gradually to find the minimum effective amount.

2. Balance THC and CBD

Patients sensitive to THC's psychoactive effects may benefit from CBD-dominant or balanced formulations.

3. Consider Method of Administration

- **Inhalation (smoking or vaping):** Rapid onset, shorter duration—helpful for acute symptoms.
- **Edibles and capsules:** Slower onset, longer-lasting—suitable for chronic symptom control.
- **Tinctures and oils:** Flexible dosing with moderate onset time.
- **Topicals:** Localized relief without systemic effects.

4. Monitor and Adjust

Track symptoms, side effects, and overall well-being to refine the treatment plan with healthcare provider support.

Conclusion

Cannabis interacts with the human body through the endocannabinoid system, influencing pain, inflammation, mood, and neurological health. For hydrocephalus patients, these effects offer potential avenues for symptom relief alongside conventional treatments. However, safe and effective use requires careful dosing, strain selection, and ongoing monitoring.

Chapter 5 – The Endocannabinoid System and Neurological Disorders

The endocannabinoid system (ECS) is one of the body's most important regulatory networks, influencing everything from pain perception to immune response and neural repair. In the context of neurological disorders, including hydrocephalus, the ECS plays a pivotal role in modulating inflammation, maintaining neural health, and supporting recovery after injury.

In recent years, research has begun to reveal how dysfunctions in this system may contribute to the progression of neurological conditions, and how cannabinoids from the cannabis plant could be harnessed to restore balance. Understanding these connections is critical for evaluating cannabis as a complementary therapy in hydrocephalus care.

The ECS in Neurological Function

The ECS is deeply embedded in the brain and central nervous system. Its activity influences:

- **Neuroprotection:** Shielding neurons from oxidative stress and excitotoxicity.
- **Synaptic Plasticity:** Supporting the brain's ability to adapt and form new connections.
- **Neuroinflammation Control:** Regulating immune cell activity in the central nervous system.
- **Cerebrovascular Function:** Affecting blood flow and, indirectly, the dynamics of cerebrospinal fluid (CSF).

Two primary receptors mediate these effects:

- **CB1 Receptors:** Concentrated in neurons, particularly in areas related to pain, memory, and movement.
- **CB2 Receptors:** Primarily found in immune cells, including those within the brain (microglia), where they regulate inflammatory responses.

ECS Dysfunction in Neurological Disorders

Emerging evidence suggests that ECS imbalances are linked to various neurological diseases, including multiple sclerosis, Alzheimer's disease, epilepsy, Parkinson's disease, and potentially hydrocephalus. In hydrocephalus specifically, dysfunction may involve:

1. Altered Neuroinflammatory Responses

Hydrocephalus often triggers inflammation due to injury, infection, or increased intracranial pressure. Overactive inflammation can worsen tissue damage. ECS signaling, particularly through CB2 receptors, helps regulate immune responses and may reduce harmful inflammation.

2. Impaired Neural Plasticity

Long-term hydrocephalus can affect brain development and adaptive capacity. Since the ECS plays a role in neurogenesis and synaptic remodeling, its dysfunction may limit recovery potential.

3. Disrupted CSF Regulation

While research is still emerging, cannabinoid receptors have been identified in areas of the brain involved in fluid regulation. ECS dysregulation could potentially influence CSF production and absorption, though more targeted studies are needed.

Cannabinoid Interactions with the ECS in Neurological Care
Cannabis-derived cannabinoids can influence ECS activity in ways that may be relevant to hydrocephalus:

THC

- Binds directly to CB1 and CB2 receptors.
- Modulates pain signaling pathways in the brain and spinal cord.
- Reduces overactive immune responses via CB2 activation.

CBD

- Indirectly boosts endocannabinoid tone by inhibiting FAAH (which breaks down anandamide).
- Reduces neuroinflammation by modulating cytokine production.
- Interacts with serotonin and TRPV1 receptors, influencing mood and pain perception.

Minor Cannabinoids and Terpenes

- Cannabigerol (CBG) shows neuroprotective and anti-inflammatory potential.
- Terpenes like myrcene and beta-caryophyllene can synergize with cannabinoids for enhanced effects—a phenomenon known as the *entourage effect*.

Relevance to Hydrocephalus

For individuals with hydrocephalus, ECS-targeted therapy could address multiple symptom domains:

- **Headache and Pain Relief:** By modulating nociceptive (pain) pathways.
- **Inflammation Control:** Particularly valuable in cases of post-surgical irritation or inflammation from secondary causes.
- **Neuroprotection:** Helping preserve brain function under chronic pressure or post-injury conditions.
- **Mood and Sleep Support:** Managing stress, anxiety, and sleep disruptions common in chronic neurological illness.

Research Insights

While direct studies on cannabis use in hydrocephalus are limited, related neurological research provides valuable insights:

- **Multiple Sclerosis (MS):** Cannabis-based medicines have been shown to reduce muscle spasticity and neuropathic pain—symptoms that share neural pathways with certain hydrocephalus-related discomforts.
- **Epilepsy:** CBD has been FDA-approved for rare seizure disorders, illustrating its ability to modulate neuronal excitability.
- **Traumatic Brain Injury (TBI):** Preclinical studies show cannabinoids can reduce neuroinflammation and protect neural tissue after injury, suggesting potential benefits for hydrocephalus cases caused by trauma.

Limitations and Areas for Further Study

Despite promising signals, significant gaps remain in the research:

- Few, if any, large-scale clinical trials have evaluated cannabis specifically for hydrocephalus.
- Long-term effects of cannabinoid use in neurological populations, especially pediatric cases, require more study.
- Individual responses vary widely, highlighting the need for personalized treatment approaches.

Clinical Considerations

When incorporating cannabis into neurological care, including hydrocephalus management:

- Work closely with healthcare providers experienced in cannabinoid therapy.
- Monitor for drug interactions with seizure medications, anti-inflammatories, or antidepressants.
- Use lab-tested products to ensure consistent dosing and safety.
- Adjust cannabinoid ratios (CBD:THC) to balance symptom relief with cognitive tolerability.

Conclusion

The endocannabinoid system is a key player in brain health, immune regulation, and neural adaptation. While direct research on cannabis in hydrocephalus is still in its infancy, evidence from related neurological disorders suggests that cannabinoids could offer valuable symptom relief and protective effects. With careful, individualized use, ECS-targeted therapies have the potential to complement traditional hydrocephalus treatments, providing a more holistic approach to care.

Chapter 6 – Scientific Research on Cannabis and Neurological Health

The therapeutic potential of cannabis in neurological conditions has attracted growing scientific interest over the last two decades. While research directly addressing hydrocephalus remains scarce, a wealth of studies on related neurological disorders—such as traumatic brain injury, multiple sclerosis, epilepsy, and neurodegenerative diseases—provides valuable insight into how cannabinoids may benefit patients facing chronic neurological challenges.

This chapter examines the most relevant scientific findings, including preclinical laboratory work, human clinical trials, and observational studies. By analyzing the mechanisms, benefits, and limitations uncovered so far, we can better understand the possible applications of cannabis-based therapies in hydrocephalus care.

Preclinical Evidence: Laying the Groundwork

Animal studies have been critical in exploring how cannabinoids interact with the brain and nervous system under stress, injury, or disease conditions. While these studies are not definitive for humans, they offer important clues.

Neuroprotection and Anti-Inflammatory Effects

- **Traumatic Brain Injury Models:** Studies have shown that cannabinoids can reduce neuroinflammation by modulating microglial cell activity and suppressing the release of pro-inflammatory cytokines. This is relevant to hydrocephalus cases resulting from trauma, where inflammation exacerbates neural damage.
- **Oxidative Stress Reduction:** Cannabinoids like CBD demonstrate strong antioxidant effects in lab settings, reducing oxidative damage that can lead to neuron death.
- **Excitotoxicity Control:** Overactivation of certain brain receptors after injury can cause further damage. THC and CBD have both been shown to help regulate glutamate release, protecting neurons from excitotoxic harm.

Cerebrovascular and CSF Flow Insights

Preclinical work has hinted that the ECS may influence cerebral blood flow and water balance in the brain. Although these findings are early, they suggest potential implications for conditions involving fluid dynamics, including hydrocephalus.

Clinical Research: Human Studies and Trials

Multiple Sclerosis (MS)

- **Nabiximols (Sativex®):** An oromucosal spray containing THC and CBD has been approved in several countries for MS-related spasticity and neuropathic pain. Multiple randomized controlled trials (RCTs) have demonstrated improvements in muscle stiffness, pain, and sleep quality.
- **Relevance to Hydrocephalus:** While MS and hydrocephalus differ in cause, both can involve spasticity, nerve pain, and mobility issues—symptoms potentially responsive to cannabinoids.

Epilepsy

- **CBD (Epidiolex®):** FDA-approved for rare seizure disorders like Dravet and Lennox-Gastaut syndromes. Multiple RCTs have shown significant seizure reduction with high-purity CBD.
- **Relevance to Hydrocephalus:** Seizures can occur in hydrocephalus, especially when there is cortical scarring or shunt-related complications. CBD's anti-seizure effects could be beneficial in select patients.

Chronic Pain Disorders

- Studies across various chronic pain conditions indicate that THC, CBD, or balanced combinations can reduce neuropathic and inflammatory pain.
- Improvements in pain often lead to better sleep, reduced anxiety, and higher quality of life—factors that can indirectly improve hydrocephalus management.

Neurodegenerative Diseases

- **Alzheimer's Disease:** Preclinical and small human studies suggest cannabinoids may slow plaque accumulation and reduce neuroinflammation.
- **Parkinson's Disease:** Small trials and surveys have reported reduced tremors, improved sleep, and reduced pain after cannabis use.
- **Relevance to Hydrocephalus:** While hydrocephalus is not neurodegenerative in the same way, the neuroprotective and anti-inflammatory mechanisms overlap.

Observational and Case Studies

Though not as scientifically rigorous as RCTs, observational studies and patient-reported outcomes provide valuable real-world perspectives:

- **Pain Relief:** Many patients report significant reductions in headache severity and frequency with cannabis use.
- **Sleep Quality:** Improvement in sleep onset and duration is a consistent finding across conditions.
- **Mood Stabilization:** Reports indicate lower anxiety levels and better emotional resilience in patients with chronic neurological illness using cannabis.

One small case series documented hydrocephalus patients who used cannabis adjunctively to traditional treatments. While anecdotal, these individuals reported reduced headaches, improved mood, and less reliance on opioid pain medications.

Limitations of the Current Research

While promising, the scientific landscape is far from complete:

- **Lack of Hydrocephalus-Specific Trials:** No large-scale, controlled studies have been conducted exclusively on hydrocephalus patients.
- **Variability in Cannabis Preparations:** Differences in cannabinoid ratios, terpene profiles, and administration routes make it difficult to compare studies.
- **Regulatory Barriers:** In many regions, legal restrictions still limit the scope and scale of cannabis research.
- **Long-Term Safety Data:** More research is needed to understand the cognitive and developmental effects of prolonged cannabinoid use, especially in pediatric patients.

Key Takeaways from the Evidence

1. **Mechanistic Overlap:** Many mechanisms by which cannabinoids benefit other neurological disorders—such as inflammation control, neuroprotection, and pain modulation—are directly relevant to hydrocephalus symptoms.
2. **Symptom-Focused Relief:** While cannabis is not a cure, it may serve as a supportive therapy to address headaches, sleep disturbances, mood changes, and inflammation.
3. **Need for Personalized Approaches:** Variability in patient response highlights the importance of individualized cannabinoid selection, dosing, and delivery method.

Conclusion

Scientific research on cannabis and neurological health supports the idea that cannabinoids can offer meaningful symptom relief and potentially protective effects for the brain. While direct hydrocephalus-specific evidence is limited, the overlap in mechanisms and symptom profiles between hydrocephalus and other neurological conditions makes this an area worth deeper exploration.

Chapter 7 – Cannabinoid Therapy Options for Hydrocephalus

Cannabinoid therapy is not a one-size-fits-all approach. For individuals living with hydrocephalus, selecting the right cannabinoids, balancing their ratios, choosing the appropriate method of administration, and setting a safe and effective dosage are crucial steps toward maximizing therapeutic benefits while minimizing potential risks.

This chapter will break down the two most well-known cannabinoids—CBD (cannabidiol) and THC (tetrahydrocannabinol)—and explore other minor cannabinoids and plant compounds that may have value. We will also address delivery methods, dosage strategies, and the importance of individualized treatment plans in hydrocephalus care.

CBD vs. THC: Understanding Their Distinct Roles

Cannabidiol (CBD)

- **Psychoactivity:** Non-psychoactive, meaning it does not produce the euphoric "high" associated with cannabis.
- **Primary Actions:** Anti-inflammatory, neuroprotective, anti-anxiety, anti-seizure.
- **Mechanisms:** Modulates the endocannabinoid system indirectly, inhibits FAAH to increase anandamide levels, interacts with serotonin and vanilloid receptors.
- **Relevance to Hydrocephalus:**
  - May reduce inflammation in brain tissue.
  - Can help control seizures when present.
  - Supports mood stability and reduces anxiety, which can accompany chronic illness.
  - Potential neuroprotective effects to help preserve brain function over time.

Tetrahydrocannabinol (THC)

- **Psychoactivity:** Psychoactive; binds directly to CB1 receptors in the brain and CB2 receptors in the immune system.
- **Primary Actions:** Analgesic, appetite stimulant, anti-nausea, muscle relaxant.
- **Mechanisms:** Alters neurotransmitter release, reduces pain perception, and modulates appetite and mood.
- **Relevance to Hydrocephalus:**
  - Can reduce chronic headaches and post-surgical pain.
  - May improve appetite and nutritional intake for patients experiencing weight loss.
  - Can support sleep when pain or anxiety interferes with rest.

Minor Cannabinoids and Their Potential Roles

Cannabigerol (CBG)

- Anti-inflammatory and neuroprotective properties.
- May help regulate intraocular pressure—relevant in patients with secondary complications involving vision.

Cannabinol (CBN)

- Mildly psychoactive.
- Often linked to sedative effects, potentially useful for sleep issues.

Tetrahydrocannabivarin (THCV)

- May modulate THC's psychoactivity.
- Potential anti-inflammatory effects.

Beta-Caryophyllene (a Terpene)

- Binds to CB2 receptors, offering anti-inflammatory effects without psychoactivity.
- Found in black pepper, cloves, and certain cannabis strains.

Balancing Cannabinoid Ratios for Hydrocephalus

The ratio of CBD to THC can significantly influence both therapeutic benefits and side effect profiles.

High-CBD, Low-THC (e.g., 20:1 or higher)

- Best for patients sensitive to THC or those seeking symptom relief without intoxication.
- Often used for inflammation, seizure control, and anxiety management.

Balanced CBD:THC (e.g., 1:1)

- Offers both anti-inflammatory and analgesic benefits.
- CBD may temper THC's psychoactive effects, allowing for better tolerability.

High-THC, Low-CBD (e.g., 5:1 or higher)

- Suitable for severe pain, appetite stimulation, and certain sleep issues.
- Should be used with caution in patients prone to anxiety or cognitive impairment.

Methods of Administration

Each method of cannabis delivery has unique benefits and limitations.

1. Inhalation (Smoking or Vaping)

- **Onset:** 1–5 minutes.
- **Duration:** 2–4 hours.
- **Advantages:** Rapid relief, easy dose titration.
- **Drawbacks:** Smoking can irritate lungs; vaping is less harsh but still not risk-free.

2. Oral Ingestion (Edibles, Capsules)

- **Onset:** 30–90 minutes.
- **Duration:** 6–8 hours or longer.
- **Advantages:** Long-lasting relief; discreet.
- **Drawbacks:** Harder to titrate dose due to delayed onset; risk of overconsumption.

3. Sublingual (Tinctures, Sprays)

- **Onset:** 15–45 minutes.
- **Duration:** 4–6 hours.
- **Advantages:** Faster onset than edibles, more precise dosing.
- **Drawbacks:** Taste may be unpleasant for some.

4. Topical (Creams, Balms, Patches)

- **Onset:** Variable (minutes to hours).
- **Duration:** Up to 8 hours.
- **Advantages:** Localized relief without systemic effects; non-intoxicating.

- **Drawbacks:** Limited to surface-level or muscle-related symptoms.

Dosing Strategies for Hydrocephalus Patients

A thoughtful dosing plan is essential, particularly for individuals new to cannabis or those with complex neurological conditions.

General Guidelines

1. **Start Low and Go Slow:** Begin with the smallest possible dose, especially with THC. Increase gradually every few days until desired effect is achieved.
2. **Track Effects:** Keep a journal of dosage, timing, and symptom changes.
3. **Be Patient:** Finding the optimal dose and ratio may take several weeks.

CBD Dosage Considerations

- Often effective at higher daily doses (20–100+ mg depending on severity of symptoms).
- Minimal side effects, though fatigue or digestive changes can occur.

THC Dosage Considerations

- Beginners may start at 1–2.5 mg THC per dose.
- Higher doses (5–10 mg) may be needed for severe pain or sleep issues, but increase risk of psychoactive effects.

Safety Considerations and Precautions

- **Medical Oversight:** Work with a healthcare provider, especially if taking other medications.
- **Drug Interactions:** Cannabinoids may alter metabolism of seizure drugs, antidepressants, and blood thinners.
- **Cognitive Sensitivity:** Patients with existing cognitive impairment should be cautious with THC.
- **Pediatric Use:** Requires strict medical supervision due to potential impacts on brain development.
- **Legal Compliance:** Ensure any cannabis use follows local laws and regulations.

Conclusion

Cannabinoid therapy offers a spectrum of options for hydrocephalus patients, from CBD-rich regimens aimed at reducing inflammation and seizures to balanced CBD:THC formulations for pain and sleep support. By tailoring cannabinoid ratios, dosing schedules, and delivery methods to individual needs, patients can achieve meaningful symptom relief while minimizing side effects.

Chapter 8 – Legal and Ethical Considerations in Cannabis Use

Cannabis laws vary widely around the world and even within individual countries, creating a complex legal landscape for patients, caregivers, and healthcare providers. For individuals with hydrocephalus considering cannabinoid therapy, understanding the legal framework and the ethical implications of use is essential—not only to ensure compliance but also to safeguard patient rights, medical integrity, and informed decision-making.

This chapter explores the current legal status of medical cannabis in key regions, the challenges of navigating differing regulations, and the ethical considerations that arise when integrating cannabis into hydrocephalus care.

1. The Global Legal Landscape

Cannabis legality falls into three broad categories: fully legal (medical and recreational use permitted), medical use only, or fully prohibited. Even within these categories, rules on cultivation, possession, and product access can differ significantly.

North America

- **United States:**
    - Federally, cannabis remains classified as a Schedule I controlled substance, meaning it is considered to have a high potential for abuse and no accepted medical use.
    - However, as of this writing, over 30 states plus the District of Columbia have legalized medical cannabis, and several have legalized recreational use.
    - State-level programs differ in qualifying conditions, purchase limits, and allowable products. Hydrocephalus may not be listed as a qualifying condition, but related symptoms such as chronic pain, seizures, or spasticity may qualify a patient.
- **Canada:**
    - Cannabis is legal nationwide for both medical and recreational purposes.
    - Patients may access cannabis through licensed producers, and medical authorization allows for higher possession limits.
- **Mexico:**
    - Medical cannabis with less than 1% THC is legal, and broader legalization measures are under development.

Europe

- **Netherlands:** Tolerates recreational use in "coffee shops" and provides medical cannabis via prescription.
- **Germany:** Legalized medical cannabis in 2017; covered by insurance in certain cases.
- **United Kingdom:** Legalized medical cannabis in 2018, but prescriptions are limited and tightly controlled.

Asia-Pacific

- **Israel:** A leader in medical cannabis research and regulation, offering access for a wide range of conditions.
- **Thailand:** Legalized medical cannabis in 2018 and has since expanded cultivation rights.
- **Australia & New Zealand:** Both have legalized medical cannabis under strict regulations, with varying product availability.

2. Legal Barriers and Access Challenges

Even where cannabis is legal for medical use, patients often face obstacles:

- **Limited Qualifying Conditions:** Hydrocephalus may not appear on official lists, requiring patients to qualify under related conditions.
- **Physician Reluctance:** Some providers may hesitate to prescribe cannabis due to stigma, lack of training, or fear of regulatory scrutiny.
- **Cost and Insurance:** In many regions, cannabis is not covered by insurance, creating a financial barrier for long-term use.
- **Product Consistency:** Variability in potency and quality between batches can make symptom management challenging without reliable suppliers.

3. Ethical Considerations in Medical Cannabis Use

a. Patient Autonomy

Patients have the right to make informed choices about their treatment options, including cannabis. This requires access to unbiased, evidence-based information and the ability to weigh potential benefits against risks.

b. Informed Consent

Healthcare providers should ensure that patients understand:

- The known and unknown effects of cannabis on hydrocephalus symptoms.
- Potential interactions with existing medications.
- The legal implications of use in their jurisdiction.

c. Clinical Responsibility

Clinicians should avoid prescribing cannabis without proper assessment, monitoring, and follow-up, even in regions where it is legally accessible.

d. Pediatric and Vulnerable Populations

Special caution is needed when prescribing to children or individuals with cognitive impairment, as the developing brain is more susceptible to the effects of cannabinoids. Ethical care includes exploring all non-risk alternatives first and using cannabis only under close medical supervision.

4. Navigating the Regulatory Environment

For Patients:

- **Know Your Local Laws:** Research your state, province, or country's cannabis regulations.
- **Register if Required:** Some jurisdictions require enrollment in a medical cannabis program for legal protection.
- **Purchase from Licensed Sources:** This ensures product quality and avoids legal penalties.

For Caregivers:

- Understand the possession and administration laws to avoid accidental violations.
- Maintain accurate records of dosing, product type, and observed effects.

For Healthcare Providers:

- Stay updated on evolving regulations to provide accurate guidance.
- Document clinical reasoning for cannabis recommendations in patient records.

5. Balancing Legal Risks and Medical Needs

For some patients, the potential benefits of cannabis—such as pain reduction, seizure control, or improved sleep—may outweigh legal concerns. However, this calculation must be made with full awareness of potential consequences:

- **Employment Risks:** Certain professions conduct regular drug testing and may not accommodate medical cannabis use.
- **Travel Restrictions:** Crossing borders with cannabis, even for medical purposes, can result in severe legal penalties.
- **Custody or Guardianship Concerns:** In some jurisdictions, cannabis use—medical or otherwise—can complicate custody cases.

6. The Future of Cannabis Regulation

Global trends suggest a gradual shift toward broader legalization, with growing emphasis on medical research, quality control, and patient access. This shift is being driven by:

- Increasing public support for medical cannabis.
- Expanding scientific evidence for therapeutic benefits.
- Recognition of cannabis as an alternative to opioids for chronic pain management.

Still, the pace of reform varies, and patients must navigate a patchwork of laws for the foreseeable future.

Conclusion

For hydrocephalus patients, the decision to use cannabis involves more than medical considerations—it is also a legal and ethical choice that must be made with clear understanding of the regulatory environment. Patients, caregivers, and healthcare providers must work together to ensure that cannabis use is compliant with the law, grounded in sound clinical judgment, and aligned with the patient's values and health goals.

Chapter 9 – Debunking Common Myths and Misconceptions About Cannabis

Despite increasing legalization and medical research, cannabis remains one of the most misunderstood therapeutic options in modern healthcare. Misinformation—rooted in decades of political propaganda, inconsistent research, and anecdotal exaggerations—continues to influence public opinion, policy decisions, and even patient care.

For individuals with hydrocephalus considering cannabis therapy, separating fact from fiction is crucial. Misconceptions can lead to unrealistic expectations, poor decision-making, or avoidance of a potentially helpful treatment.

This chapter addresses some of the most persistent myths about cannabis, replacing them with accurate, evidence-based insights.

1. Myth: "Cannabis Has No Medical Value"

Reality:

- This claim dates back to the early-to-mid 20th century when cannabis was classified as a Schedule I drug in the U.S., implying it had "no accepted medical use."
- Modern research, however, has documented cannabis's benefits for conditions such as chronic pain, chemotherapy-induced nausea, multiple sclerosis spasticity, and certain seizure disorders.
- While hydrocephalus-specific studies are limited, the symptom overlap (e.g., pain, headaches, muscle spasticity, sleep disturbances) suggests a clear potential role for cannabis in symptom management.

2. Myth: "Cannabis Use Always Leads to Addiction"

Reality:

- Cannabis can cause dependence, but the risk is lower than that of alcohol, nicotine, or opioids.
- The National Institute on Drug Abuse estimates that about 9% of cannabis users develop dependence—compared to 15% for alcohol and 32% for nicotine.
- Risk increases with heavy, long-term, recreational use, particularly when initiated in adolescence.
- For medical patients using controlled doses under supervision, the risk of addiction is significantly lower.

3. Myth: "Cannabis Will Make You 'High' No Matter What"

Reality:

- Not all cannabis products cause psychoactive effects. The primary intoxicating compound is **tetrahydrocannabinol (THC)**, but other cannabinoids such as **cannabidiol (CBD)** are non-intoxicating.
- Medical formulations can be tailored to minimize THC or balance it with CBD to reduce or eliminate unwanted psychoactivity.
- Topicals, suppositories, and certain microdoses can provide therapeutic benefits without noticeable intoxication.

4. Myth: "Smoking is the Only Way to Use Cannabis"

Reality:

- Inhaling cannabis smoke is only one of many delivery methods—and often not the healthiest.
- Alternatives include:
    - **Vaporization:** Reduces combustion-related toxins.
    - **Oils and Tinctures:** Sublingual absorption for quick onset.
    - **Capsules and Edibles:** Long-lasting effects but slower onset.
    - **Topicals:** Localized relief without systemic psychoactive effects.
    - **Transdermal Patches:** Steady cannabinoid delivery over hours.

5. Myth: "Cannabis is a Cure-All"

Reality:

- Cannabis is not a miracle cure. It may alleviate symptoms but rarely addresses the root cause of a condition.
- For hydrocephalus, cannabis cannot replace shunt surgery or other conventional interventions—it is best used as part of a comprehensive treatment plan.
- Overstating cannabis's potential can lead to disappointment, delay in necessary medical care, and distrust in legitimate cannabis research.

6. Myth: "Cannabis Kills Brain Cells"

Reality:

- This myth originated from flawed animal studies in the 1970s that have since been discredited.
- Recent research suggests cannabinoids may actually have **neuroprotective** properties, reducing oxidative stress and inflammation in the brain.
- That said, heavy THC exposure during adolescence may affect brain development—reinforcing the need for careful medical oversight.

7. Myth: "Medical Cannabis is the Same as Street Cannabis"

Reality:

- Medical cannabis is cultivated, processed, and tested under strict quality control to ensure consistent cannabinoid content and the absence of contaminants like pesticides, mold, or heavy metals.
- Street cannabis is unregulated, with unknown potency and purity, increasing the risk of unpredictable effects or harmful exposure.

8. Myth: "CBD Alone is Enough for All Medical Needs"

Reality:

- While CBD offers anti-inflammatory, anti-anxiety, and anti-seizure benefits, some conditions respond better to a combination of cannabinoids—a phenomenon known as the **entourage effect**.
- For hydrocephalus-related symptoms, balanced THC:CBD ratios may be more effective for pain, muscle spasticity, or nausea than CBD alone.

9. Myth: "Cannabis Laws Are the Same Everywhere"

Reality:

- Cannabis legality varies not only from country to country but also between states, provinces, or even cities.
- Patients must research and comply with local laws to avoid legal consequences.
- Assuming legality in one area applies everywhere can lead to severe penalties, especially when traveling internationally.

10. Myth: "Cannabis is Harmless"

Reality:

- While safer than many pharmaceuticals in terms of overdose risk, cannabis can still cause side effects—dry mouth, dizziness, increased heart rate, or anxiety—especially with high THC doses.
- Potential interactions with other medications must be considered.
- Certain populations (e.g., pregnant women, adolescents, individuals with psychiatric conditions) require extra caution.

Why Dispelling Myths Matters for Hydrocephalus Patients
Misinformation can result in:

- **Missed Opportunities:** Patients avoiding cannabis due to stigma or fear.
- **Unsafe Use:** Improper dosing, unsafe sourcing, or neglect of conventional treatment.
- **Policy Stagnation:** Legislators and healthcare systems resisting reform due to outdated beliefs.

By addressing myths head-on, patients, caregivers, and healthcare providers can create an informed, stigma-free environment that allows cannabis to be considered objectively—based on scientific evidence and patient needs rather than hearsay or propaganda.

Conclusion
Understanding the truths behind cannabis is essential for making responsible medical decisions, especially for those managing complex neurological conditions like hydrocephalus. Dispelling myths is not about promoting cannabis blindly—it's about creating clarity so that patients can weigh the benefits and risks without the cloud of misinformation.

Chapter 10 – Practical Guidelines for Integrating Cannabis into Hydrocephalus Care

Cannabis can be a valuable complementary therapy for individuals living with hydrocephalus, but its benefits are maximized—and risks minimized—when used thoughtfully, strategically, and under professional guidance. Because hydrocephalus is a complex neurological condition with varying causes, severities, and treatment histories, cannabis use must be tailored to each patient's unique needs.

This chapter provides a comprehensive roadmap for integrating cannabis into hydrocephalus care, including patient assessment, product selection, dosing, monitoring, and ongoing care adjustments.

1. Initial Considerations Before Starting Cannabis

a. Medical Clearance

- Consult with a neurologist, neurosurgeon, or primary care physician who understands both hydrocephalus and cannabis pharmacology.
- Discuss potential interactions with existing medications, particularly anticonvulsants, anti-nausea drugs, pain medications, and any blood thinners.

b. Legal Compliance

- Research the specific laws in your state, province, or country regarding medical cannabis access, possession limits, and qualifying conditions.
- Obtain the necessary medical documentation or patient registration if required by local regulations.

c. Setting Goals

- Identify your therapeutic priorities (e.g., pain reduction, nausea control, improved sleep, anxiety relief).
- Establish measurable goals, such as reducing headache intensity by a certain percentage or improving sleep duration.

2. Choosing the Right Cannabis Products

a. Cannabinoid Ratios

- **High-CBD, Low-THC** formulations: Ideal for reducing inflammation, mild pain, or anxiety without psychoactive effects.
- **Balanced THC:CBD Ratios** (e.g., 1:1 or 2:1): May offer more robust pain and spasticity relief while limiting intoxication.
- **THC-Dominant**: Reserved for patients with high tolerance or severe symptoms unresponsive to lower THC options; should be approached with caution.

b. Delivery Methods

- **Tinctures/Oils (Sublingual)**: Fast onset (15–45 minutes) and easy to titrate dosage.
- **Capsules/Softgels**: Discreet, pre-measured doses with slower onset (1–2 hours) but longer-lasting effects.
- **Vaporization**: Rapid relief for breakthrough symptoms, but less suitable for patients with respiratory conditions.
- **Topicals**: Best for localized pain (e.g., neck stiffness, shunt site tenderness).
- **Edibles**: Long-lasting effects, but dose control is more difficult—start low to avoid overconsumption.

3. Dosing Strategies for Hydrocephalus Patients

a. The "Start Low, Go Slow" Principle

- Begin with the smallest possible effective dose, particularly if new to cannabis.
- Gradually increase dose every 3–5 days until desired symptom relief is achieved, avoiding large jumps in dosage.

b. Microdosing

- Using very small amounts (1–2 mg THC or CBD) throughout the day can provide symptom relief without sedation or intoxication.
- Particularly useful for managing chronic symptoms such as headache or mood fluctuations.

c. Symptom-Specific Adjustments

- **For Headaches:** Balanced THC:CBD tinctures or vaporization for fast relief.
- **For Muscle Spasms:** Slightly higher THC ratios may help reduce spasticity.
- **For Anxiety/Insomnia:** High-CBD products in the daytime; THC-inclusive options in the evening for sleep.

4. Integrating Cannabis with Conventional Hydrocephalus Treatments

a. Post-Surgical Recovery

- Cannabis should not replace prescribed post-operative medications unless approved by the surgical team.
- May be used to complement pain control and reduce reliance on opioids.

b. Shunt-Related Symptoms

- Cannabis may help alleviate discomfort at the shunt site, muscle tension in the neck, or anxiety related to shunt revisions.

c. Cognitive Function Monitoring

- Some hydrocephalus patients experience cognitive challenges—care should be taken to avoid high-THC doses that could temporarily worsen short-term memory or focus.

5. Safety and Monitoring Protocols

a. Side Effect Awareness

- Common: Dry mouth, mild dizziness, increased appetite, drowsiness.
- Less common but possible: Anxiety, rapid heart rate, confusion (often from excessive THC).

b. Regular Check-Ins

- Maintain a symptom journal tracking cannabis dose, product type, time of use, and symptom relief.
- Schedule follow-up appointments every 4–8 weeks with your healthcare provider to assess progress.

c. Interaction Management

- Cannabis can interact with medications metabolized by the liver's **CYP450 enzyme system**—dosage adjustments to either cannabis or other medications may be necessary.

6. Lifestyle and Holistic Integration

a. Pairing with Non-Pharmacological Strategies

- Gentle stretching, mindfulness meditation, adequate hydration, and dietary adjustments can enhance cannabis's therapeutic effects.

b. Emotional Support

- Engage in counseling or patient support groups to address emotional and psychological challenges alongside physical symptoms.

c. Long-Term Sustainability

- Periodically reassess whether cannabis remains the best therapeutic choice, as tolerance, symptoms, or legal access may change over time.

7. Red Flags – When to Seek Medical Attention

- Sudden worsening of headaches, vision changes, or balance issues (possible shunt malfunction).
- Severe confusion, agitation, or hallucinations after cannabis use.
- Allergic reactions (rash, swelling, difficulty breathing).

Conclusion

Cannabis integration for hydrocephalus patients is a highly personalized process. Success lies in careful product selection, gradual dosing, symptom monitoring, and maintaining open communication with healthcare providers. By approaching cannabis as a strategic, data-driven component of care—rather than a quick fix—patients can safely explore its potential benefits while preserving overall neurological health.

Appendix A – Cannabis Strain and Product Reference for Hydrocephalus Symptom Management

This appendix serves as a quick-reference guide for patients, caregivers, and healthcare providers looking to match specific hydrocephalus symptoms with cannabis-based solutions. It is designed to help users make informed choices while collaborating with medical professionals and dispensary specialists.

The strains and product categories listed here are examples based on current research, patient reports, and clinical insights. Individual responses to cannabis vary, so what works well for one person may be less effective for another.

1. Symptom-to-Product Matching Table

Symptom / Challenge	Recommended Cannabinoid Profile	Potential Strains / Product Examples	Preferred Delivery Methods	Notes & Cautions
Chronic Headaches & Intracranial Pressure Discomfort	Balanced THC:CBD (1:1 or 2:1)	Harlequin, Cannatonic, Pennywise	Tincture, Vaporizer	Start with low doses; high THC may worsen pressure headaches in sensitive users
Muscle Spasms / Neck Tension (often near shunt site)	Moderate THC (10–15%) + CBD	Blueberry, ACDC, Sour Tsunami	Tincture, Capsule, Topical	Topicals can target local muscle tightness without systemic effects
Anxiety / Mood Swings	High CBD, low THC (<5%)	Charlotte's Web, Ringo's Gift	Tincture, Capsule	Avoid strong sativa THC strains if anxiety-prone

Symptom / Challenge	Recommended Cannabinoid Profile	Potential Strains / Product Examples	Preferred Delivery Methods	Notes & Cautions
Sleep Difficulties	THC-dominant indica with sedative terpenes	Granddaddy Purple, Northern Lights	Tincture (evening), Edible	Test on non-work nights first to monitor sedation levels
Nausea / Appetite Loss	THC-forward (10–20%) with uplifting terpenes	Durban Poison, Maui Wowie	Vaporizer, Capsule	Vaporization offers fastest nausea relief
Post-Surgical Pain	Balanced or THC-forward	OG Kush, White Widow	Tincture, Capsule, Topical	Use topicals for localized incision site relief
Cognitive Fog	CBD-dominant (15%+) with minimal THC	Suzy Q, Elektra	Tincture, Capsule	Excess THC may temporarily impair memory
Emotional Distress / Depression	Balanced or slightly sativa-leaning	Jack Herer, Canna-Tsu	Tincture, Vaporizer	Use with caution; energizing strains may interfere with sleep if taken late

2. Understanding Terpenes and Their Role

Beyond cannabinoids like THC and CBD, terpenes—the aromatic compounds in cannabis—play an important role in symptom relief.

Terpene	Potential Benefits for Hydrocephalus Patients	Common in Strains
Myrcene	Sedative, muscle relaxant, pain relief	Granddaddy Purple, Blue Dream
Linalool	Calming, anti-anxiety, anti-inflammatory	Lavender Kush, Amnesia Haze
Limonene	Mood elevation, anti-anxiety	Super Lemon Haze, Durban Poison
Beta-Caryophyllene	Anti-inflammatory, pain relief, gut support	Girl Scout Cookies, Bubba Kush
Pinene	Improves focus, reduces inflammation	Jack Herer, Harlequin

3. Product Formulation Recommendations

- **Tinctures & Oils** – Best for consistent daily dosing and discreet use. Can be taken sublingually for faster absorption.
- **Capsules** – Provide precise dosing; slower onset but longer-lasting effects.
- **Vaporization** – Fastest relief; useful for breakthrough symptoms but less suitable for long-term daily use due to respiratory concerns.
- **Edibles** – Provide extended symptom coverage but require careful dose control to avoid overconsumption.
- **Topicals** – Best for localized discomfort without psychoactive effects; useful around muscle tension near shunt areas.

4. Safe Dosing Reference

Experience Level	THC Starting Dose	CBD Starting Dose	Notes
Beginner / Sensitive	1–2 mg THC	5–10 mg CBD	Wait at least 6 hours before re-dosing
Intermediate	2.5–5 mg THC	10–20 mg CBD	Increase by 1–2 mg as needed every 3–5 days
Experienced / Tolerant	5–10 mg THC	20–40 mg CBD	Maintain lowest effective dose to avoid tolerance buildup

5. Cautions and Contraindications

- Avoid driving or operating machinery until you understand how cannabis affects you.
- Monitor for increased confusion, dizziness, or balance issues—these can be exacerbated by cannabis in hydrocephalus patients.
- Use caution with THC if you have a history of psychosis or severe anxiety.
- Avoid combining cannabis with alcohol or sedatives without medical guidance.
- Always store products securely, away from children and pets.

6. Record-Keeping Template
Patient Cannabis Use Log

Date	Product Name / Strain	THC %	CBD %	Dose (mg)	Time Taken	Symptom(s) Targeted	Relief Rating (0–10)	Side Effects	Notes

Maintaining a record allows you and your healthcare provider to fine-tune your cannabis regimen over time.

Closing Notes
Appendix A is not intended to replace medical advice—it is a structured reference to assist in informed decision-making. By understanding cannabinoid ratios, terpene profiles, dosing strategies, and symptom-specific targeting, hydrocephalus patients and caregivers can approach cannabis integration with confidence and precision.

<u>Message from the Author:</u>

I hope you enjoyed this book, I love astrology and knew there was not a book such as this out on the shelf. I love metaphysical items as well. Please check out my other books:

-Life of Government Benefits

-My life of Hell

-My life with Hydrocephalus

-Red Sky

-World Domination:Woman's rule

-World Domination:Woman's Rule 2: The War

-Life and Banishment of Apophis: book 1

-The Kidney Friendly Diet

-The Ultimate Hemp Cookbook

-Creating a Dispensary(legally)

-Cleanliness throughout life: the importance of showering from childhood to adulthood.

-Strong Roots: The Risks of Overcoddling children

-Hemp Horoscopes: Cosmic Insights and Earthly Healing

- Celestial Hemp Navigating the Zodiac: Through the Green Cosmos

-Astrological Hemp: Aligning The Stars with Earth's Ancient Herb

-The Astrological Guide to Hemp: Stars, Signs, and Sacred Leaves

-Green Growth: Innovative Marketing Strategies for your Hemp Products and Dispensary

-Cosmic Cannabis

-Astrological Munchies

-Henry The Hemp

-Zodiacal Roots: The Astrological Soul Of Hemp

- **Green Constellations: Intersection of Hemp and Zodiac**

-Hemp in The Houses: An astrological Adventure Through The Cannabis Galaxy

-Galactic Ganja Guide
Heavenly Hemp
Zodiac Leaves
Doctor Who Astrology
Cannastrology
Stellar Satvias and Cosmic Indicas
Celestial Cannabis: A Zodiac Journey
AstroHerbology: The Sky and The Soil: Volume 1
AstroHerbology:Celestial Cannabis:Volume 2
Cosmic Cannabis Cultivation
The Starry Guide to Herbal Harmony: Volume 1
The Starry Guide to Herbal Harmony: Cannabis Universe: Volume 2
Yugioh Astrology: Astrological Guide to Deck, Duels and more
Nightmare Mansion: Echoes of The Abyss
Nightmare Mansion 2: Legacy of Shadows
Nightmare Mansion 3: Shadows of the Forgotten
Nightmare Mansion 4: Echoes of the Damned
The Life and Banishment of Apophis: Book 2
Nightmare Mansion: Halls of Despair
Healing with Herb: Cannabis and Hydrocephalus
Planetary Pot: Aligning with Astrological Herbs: Volume 1
Fast Track to Freedom: 30 Days to Financial Independence Using AI, Assets, and Agile Hustles
Cosmic Hemp Pathways
How to Become Financially Free in 30 Days: 10,000 Paths to Prosperity
Zodiacal Herbage: Astrological Insights: Volume 1
Nightmare Mansion: Whispers in the Walls
The Daleks Invade Atlantis
Henry the hemp and Hydrocephalus

10X The Kidney Friendly Diet

Cannabis Universe: Adult coloring book

Hemp Astrology: The Healing Power of the Stars

Zodiacal Herbage: Astrological Insights: Cannabis Universe: Volume 2

<u>**Planetary Pot: Aligning with Astrological Herbs: Cannabis Universes: Volume 2**</u>

Doctor Who: Convergence Protocol – The Replicator War

Nightmare Mansion: Curse of the Blood Moon

<u>**The Celestial Stoner: A Guide to the Zodiac**</u>

Cosmic Pleasures: Sex Toy Astrology for Every Sign

Hydrocephalus Astrology: Navigating the Stars and Healing Waters

Lapis and the Mischievous Chocolate Bar

Celestial Positions: Sexual Astrology for Every Sign

Apophis's Shadow Work Journal: : A Journey of Self-Discovery and Healing

Kinky Cosmos: Sexual Kink Astrology for Every Sign

Digital Cosmos: The Astrological Digimon Compendium

Stellar Seeds: The Cosmic Guide to Growing with Astrology

Apophis's Daily Gratitude Journal

Cat Astrology: Feline Mysteries of the Cosmos

The Cosmic Kama Sutra: An Astrological Guide to Sexual Positions

Unleash Your Potential: A Guided Journal Powered by AI Insights

Whispers of the Enchanted Grove

Cosmic Pleasures: An Astrological Guide to Sexual Kinks

369, 12 Manifestation Journal

Whisper of the nocturne journal(blank journal for writing or drawing)

The Boogey Book

Locked In Reflection: A Chastity Journey Through Locktober

Generating Wealth Quickly:How to Generate $100,000 in 24 Hours

Star Magic: Harness the Power of the Universe

The Flatulence Chronicles: A Fart Journal for Self-Discovery

The Doctor and The Death Moth

Seize the Day: A Personal Seizure Tracking Journal

The Ultimate Boogeyman Safari: A Journey into the Boogie World and Beyond

Whispers of Samhain: 1,000 Spells of Love, Luck, and Lunar Magic: Samhain Spell Book

Apophis's guides:Witch's Spellbook Crafting Guide for Halloween

<u>Frost & Flame: The Enchanted Yule Grimoire of 1000 Winter Spells</u>

<u>The Ultimate Boogey Goo Guide & Spooky Activities for Halloween Fun</u>

Harmony of the Scales: A Libra's Spellcraft for Balance and Beauty

The Enchanted Advent: 36 Days of Christmas Wonders

Nightmare Mansion: The Labyrinth of Screams

Harvest of Enchantment: 1,000 Spells of Gratitude, Love, and Fortune for Thanksgiving

The Boogey Chronicles: A Journal of Nightly Encounters and Shadowy Secrets

The 12 Days of Financial Freedom: A Step-by-Step Christmas Countdown to Transform Your Finances

Sigil of the Eternal Spiral Blank Journal

A Christmas Feast: Timeless Recipes for Every Meal

Holiday Stress-Free Solutions: A Survival Guide to Thriving During the Festive Season

Whispers of the Harvest: The Corn Mother's Journal

The Evergreen Spellbook

The Doctor Meets the Boogeyman

The White Witch of Rose Hall's SpellBook

The Gingerbread Golem's Shadow: A Study in Sweet Darkness

The Gingerbread Golem Codex: An Academic Exploration of Sweet Myths

The Gingerbread Golem Grimoire: Sweet Magicks and Spells for the Festive Witch

The Curse of the Gingerbread Golem

10-minute Christmas Crafts for kids

<u>Christmas Crisis Solutions: The Ultimate Last-Minute Survival Guide</u>

Gingerbread Golem Recipes: Holiday Treats with a Magical Twist

The Infinite Key: Unlocking Mystical Secrets of the Ages

Enchanted Yule: A Wiccan and Pagan Guide to a Magical and Memorable Season

Dinosaurs of Power: Unlocking Ancient Magick

Astro-Dinos: The Cosmic Guide to Prehistoric Wisdom

Gallifrey's Yule Logs: A Festive Doctor Who Cookbook

The Dino Grimoire: Secrets of Prehistoric Magick

The Gift They Never Knew They Needed

The Gingerbread Golem's Culinary Alchemy: Enchanting Recipes for a Sweetly Dark Feast

A Time Lord Christmas: Holiday Adventures with the Doctor

Krampusproofing Your Home: Defensive Strategies for Yule

Silent Frights: A Collection of Christmas Creepypastas to Chill Your Bones

Santa Raptor's Jolly Carnage: A Dino-Claus Christmas Tale

Prehistoric Palettes: A Dino Wicca Coloring Journey

The Christmas Wishkeeper Chronicles

The Starlight Sleigh: A Holiday Journey

Elf Secrets: The True Magic of the North Pole

Reclaiming Time: How to Live More by Doing Less

Chronovore: The Eternal Nexus

The Mind Reset: Unlocking Your Inner Peace in a Chaotic World

Confidence Code: Building Unshakable Self-Belief

Baby the Vampire Terrier

Baby the Vampire Terrier's Christmas Adventure

Celestial Streams: The Content Creator's Astrology Manual

The Wealth Whisperer: Unlocking Abundance with Everyday Actions

The Energy Equation: Maximize Your Output Without Burning Out

The Happiness Algorithm: Science-Backed Steps to Joyful Living

Stress-Free Success: Achieving Goals Without Anxiety

Mindful Wealth: The New Blueprint for Financial Freedom

The Festive Flavors of New Year: A Culinary Celebration

The Master's Gambit: Keys of Eternal Power

Shadowed Secrets: Groundhog Day Mysteries

Beneath the Burrow: Lessons from the Groundhog

Spring's Whispers: The Groundhog's Prediction

The Limitless Mindset: Unlock Your Untapped Potential

The Focus Funnel: How to Cut Through Chaos and Get Results

Bold Moves: Building Courage to Live on Your Terms

The Daily Shift: Simple Practices for Lasting Transformation

The Quarter-Life Reset: Thriving in Your 20s and 30s

The Art of Shadowplay: Building Your Own Personal Myth

The Eternal Loop: Finding Purpose in Repetition

Burrowing Wisdom: Life Lessons from the Groundhog

Shadow Work: A Groundhog Day Perspective

Love in Bloom: 5-Minute Romantic Gestures

The Shadowspell Codex: Secrets of Forbidden Magick

The Burnout Cure: Finding Balance in a Busy World

The Groundhog Prophecy: Unlocking Seasonal Secrets

Nog Tales: The Spirited History of Eggnog

Six More Weeks: Embracing Seasonal Transitions
The Lumivian Chronicles: Fragments of the Fifth Dimension
Money on Your Mind: A Beginner's Guide to Wealth
The Focus Fix: Breaking Through Distraction
January's Spirit Keepers: Mystical Protectors of the Cold
Creativity Unchained: Unlocking Your Wildest Ideas in 2025
Manifestation Mastery: 365 Days to Rewrite Your Reality
The Groundhog's Mirror: Reflecting on Change
The Weeping Angels' Christmas Curse
Burrowed in Time: A Groundhog Day Journey
Heartbeats: Poems to Share with Your Valentine
Dino Wicca: The Sacred Grimoire of Prehistoric Magick
Courage of the Pride: Finding Your Inner Roar
The Lion's Leap: Bold Moves for Big Results
Healthy Hustle: Achieving Without Overworking
Practical Manifesting: Turning Dreams into Reality in 2025
Jurassic Pharaohs: Unlocking the Magick of Ancient Egypt and Dino Wicca
The Happiness Equation: Small Changes for Big Joy
The Confidence Compass: Finding Your Inner Strength
Whispers in the Hollow: Tales of the Forgotten Beasts
Echoes from the Hollow: The Return of Forgotten Beasts
The Hollow Ascendant: The Rise of the Forgotten Beasts
The Relationship Reset: Building Better Connections
Mastering the Morning: How to Win the Day Before 8 AM
The Shadow's Dance: Groundhog Day Symbolism
Cupid's Kitchen: Quick Valentine's Day Recipes
Valentine's Day on a Budget: Love Without Breaking the Bank
Astrocraft: Aligning the Stars in the World of Minecraft
Forecasting Life: Groundhog Day Reflections
Bleeding Hearts: Twisted Tales of Valentine's Terror
Herbal Smoke Revolution: The Ultimate Guide to Nature's Cigarette Alternative

Winter's Wrath: The Complete Survival Blueprint for Extreme Freezes.

The Groundhog's Shadow: A Tale of Seasons

Burrowed Insights: Wisdom from the Groundhog

Sensual Strings: The Art of Erotic Bondage

Whispered Flames: Unlocking the Power of Fire Play

Forgotten Shadows: A Guide to Cryptids Lost to Time

Six Weeks of Secrets: Groundhog Day's Hidden Messages

Shadows and Cycles: Groundhog Day Reflections

The Art of Love Letters: Crafting the Perfect Message

Romantic Getaways at Home: Turning Your Space into Paradise

Purrfect Brews: A Cat Lover's Guide to Coffee and Companionship

The Groundhog's Wisdom: Timeless Lessons for Modern Life

The Shadow Oracle: Groundhog Day as a Predictor

Emerging from the Burrow: A Journey of Renewal

The Language of Love: Learning Your Partner's Love Style

Authorpreneur: The Ultimate Blueprint for Writing, Publishing, and Thriving as an Author

Weathering the Seasons: Groundhog Day Perspectives

Valentine's Day Magic: A Guide to Romantic Rituals

The Shadow Chronicles: Stories of Groundhog Day

Love and Laughter: Fun Games for Valentine's Day

AstroRealty: Unlocking the Stars for Property Success

The Groundhog's Path: A Guide to Seasonal Balance

Groundhog Day Diaries: Reflections in the Shadow

The Groundhog's Light: Illuminating the Path Ahead

Valentine's Traditions from Around the World

AI Wealth Revolution: Unlocking the Trillionaire Mindset

Love Rekindled: Reigniting Passion in Relationships

Single and Thriving: Self-Love on Valentine's Day

Emerald Legends: Mystical Tales of Ireland

Green Alchemy: Harnessing Nature's Magic

The Hearts of Horror: A Valentine's Day Nightmare

The Leprechaun's Guide to Wealth and Wisdom

Dancing with the Sidhe: Celebrating the Otherworld

Shamrocks and Shadows: Mysteries of the Green Isle

Emerald Energy: Harnessing Luck and Growth

The Gingerbread Golem's Valentine: A Sweetheart's Guide to Love and Enchantment

The Celtic Knot: Weaving Life and Destiny

Green Fire: Elemental Magic for St. Patrick's Day

Clover Chronicles: Finding Your Inner Luck

Ireland's Mystical Creatures: A Field Guide

Gingerbread Golem's Love Almanac

Prowl and Thrive: The Lion's Guide to Success

Love Alchemy: Transforming Your Life Through Heart Energy

WORLD DOMINATION: Woman's Rule 3:The New Life

The Midnight Rose: A Guide to Lunar Love Spells

The Forbidden Letters: Writing Your Own Love Prophecy

Luck and Lore: St. Patrick's Day for Modern Mystics

The Green Path: A Pagan Celebration of Renewal

The Dark Architect's Guide to Reprogramming Reality

Prankster's Paradise: A Guide to Harmless Hijinks

Manifest Your Reality: The Law of Attraction Simplified

The TARDIS Owner's Manual: Understanding the Doctor's Ship: *A complete guide to the TARDIS, its technology, secrets, and mysteries*

Starlit Romance: Astrology Secrets for Finding True Love

The Time Lord's Atlas: A Complete Guide to the Whoniverse: *A breakdown of the locations, planets, and dimensions explored in Doctor Who*

Sweetheart Shadows: The Dark Side of Love and Attraction

February Fire: Reigniting Passion in Every Area of Life

The Self-Love Toolkit: 5 Ways to Embrace Who You Are
February Sparks: Ignite Your Dreams in 28 Days
March to Success: A 31-Day Action Blueprint
Ancient Paths: The 13 Sacred Principles of Dino Wicca
Echoes of Tomorrow: Navigating the AI Revolution
The Wellness Blueprint: Balancing Mind, Body, and Soul
Green Horizons: Sustainable Living for a Better Tomorrow
The AI Wealth Code: How to Make Millions with Automation
AI-Powered Creativity: Writing, Art, and Music for Profit
Extinction Rites: Rebirthing Your Soul Through Prehistoric Magick
Sacred Serpents tarot
Celestial Enchantment blank journal
Star Strains
Culinary Journeys: Exploring Global Flavors at Home
The Hollowvale Curse
The Hollowvale Harvest
The Egg of Transformation: Awakening Your Inner Power
Blooming Into Power: A Wiccan Guide to Spring Awakening
The Nightmare Nexus: The Third Doctor's Perilous Haunting
Digital Detox: Reclaiming Your Life in a Connected World
Ostara's Path: Walking the Spiral of Renewal
The Sacred Hare
Financial Freedom: Building Wealth in the Modern Age
Spring's Cauldron: Stirring the Waters of Change
The Hollowvale Pact
Quantum Consciousness: The Science of Reality Shifting
The Hollowvale Hunger
The Sacred Waters Within: A Witch's Guide to Hydrocephalus Magick
The Raven's Nest: Building a Life of Unshakable Stability
AI and the Human Mind: The Future of Intelligence
The Hollowvale Reckoning

The Witch's Guide to Parenting: Raising Empowered and Intuitive Children

The Magick of Motherhood: Reclaiming Your Power Through Rituals

The Pagan Path to Self-Love: A Goddess's Guide to Worth and Confidence

Wild Woman Magick: Unleashing Your Primal Power

The Money Magnet Blueprint: Unlocking Unlimited Wealth

Biohacking 101: Unlock Your Body's Full Potential

The Wild Father: A Pagan Guide to Strength and Wisdom

The Sacred Masculine: Unlocking Your Inner Power

The Druid's Compass

The Warrior's Mindset

The Father's Fire

Odin's Path

Ancestral Bonds

The House That Whispers

The Magician's Code

The Wild Hunt

The Green Man's Path

The Altar of Success

The Shadow and the Sword

The High Priestess's Guide to Energy Healing

The Lunar Mother

The Sacred Self-Care Grimoire

The Womb Wisdom Codex

The Wheel of the Mother

The Witch's Guide to Manifestation

The Q2 Reset

The Ultimate Guide to AI-Powered Passive Income

Escape the 9-5

AI Feline Fortunes

The Tear-Stained Grimoire

Razorblade Runes
Cemetery Sirens
The Midnight Wristwatch
The Town That Forgets
AI Horror & Creepypasta
The Hollow Frequency
The Breach Echo
The Quiet Between Worlds
The Sigil of Tharan-Khul
Summon the Vault of Y'ha'ten
The Becoming Codex
The Profit of Az'ra-nar
The Drowned Logos
Echoes of the Eldritch Will
The Deep Ledger
Necronomicon of Networth
Covenant of the Wealthwyrm
The Whisperer's Manifesto
The Rites of Azh-K'luth
The Ark of the Crawling Coin
The Tithe of Shadows
Inkheart Abyss
The Timewinds of Y'ha-nthlei
The Spiral Labyrinth of Azag-Nirrh
The Gallifreyan Heresy of the Black Pharaoh
The Psalms of Nyog-Sotha
Black Rain Alchemy
The Infinite Maw
The Entropic Blueprint
The Oracle of Sh'guul
The Book of Breach
The Drowned Saint's Testament
Dreamcraft of the Sleeper God

The Silence Market
Cthonomics: The Dark Wealth Algorithm
Invocation of the Ten-Eyed King
Wealthbound to the Wyrm Below
Become the Unnameable
Codex of the Sovereign Flame
Rituals of Relentless Becoming
The Shadow Ascends
The Eyes Beneath You
The Will That Wakes Worlds
Silence Is a Weapon
The Mirror That Screams
The Whisper Between Moments
The Mind That Devours Fear
The Myth of the Finished Self
The Architect of Your Madness
The Voice You've Buried
The Discipline of Madness
Stormborn: Awakening Your Inner Tempest
The Mind That Ate Time
Unbind Your Becoming
The Pact You Owe Yourself
The Devourer's Diet
The Acid That Carves the Path
The Tower You Must Burn
The Breath Between Worlds
Speak Like the Deep
The Labyrinth Within
The Spine of the Sea God
Rejection Is a Portal
The Crown You Refused
The Scar Is the Spell
The Lightless Flame

The Habit of Becoming Horrific

ChickenJockey Chaos

The Gatekeeper Within

You Are Not Your Name

The Compass of the Mad

The Archive of Unsent Letters

What the Mirror Can't Show You

The Knife You Needed

Worship Nothing, Become Everything

The Other Voice

The Body the World Forgot

The Vein of the Void

The Black Bone Codex

The Puzzle of the Hidden Self (Millennium Puzzle)

The Eye That Sees the Lie *(Millennium Eye)*

The Ring of Return (Millennium Ring)

The Rod of Relentless Will *(Millennium Rod)*

The Tally of the Soul (Millennium Tauk/Necklace)

The Key to the Locked Timeline (Millennium Key)

The Scale of Sacred Decisions (Millennium Scales)

Inferno Bites: The UnOfficial Minecraft Lava Cookbook

Rot in the Attic

Prana: The Hidden Force of Your Infinite Self

The Shadow Realm Within: Transforming Darkness Into Destiny

The Borderland Collapse

Claws of Protection: Bastet's Defensive Magick

Mr. Ring-a-Ding's Madness

Yugioh Astrology: Celestial Deckcraft and Duel Destiny (2026–2027 Edition)

The Seal You Signed: Unlocking the Power You Once Feared

The Puzzle of Infinite Minds: Unlocking the Mentalism Hidden Within

Harnessed Minds: Breaking Free from Mental Control

The Eyes in the Smoke

Rootwake: The Carbon Covenant

Skitter Logic: Unlearning the Fear That Built You

Doctor Who: The World That Froths

Rootwake: The Fizz That Rewrites Flesh

Rootwake: Frothfather of the World

The Holly Pact: Blood Beneath the Mistletoe

The 2nd Mass Principle: Building Unbreakable Tribes

Web of Wits: A Survival Guide to Encounters with Anasi the Spider (Aunt Nancy)

The Hexbreaking Handbook: Effective Spells to Remove Curses

Pop Alchemy: Transform Your Life One Sip at a Time

The Mason Code: Leading in Unleadable Times

Petosiris and the Fifth Chamber of Thoth

The Ether Seed Within

The Parent of Tomorrow

Petosiris's Pyramid of Perpetual Wealth

Unlearn the World

Grimoire of the Hollow Tongue

Zodiac Weeds: Finding Your Strain Through the Stars

Aquarius Rises in the Bank

The Sugar God's Smile

The Skinclock Reversal: Biohacking the Face of Time

Debtburn: How to Obliterate What You Owe Forever

The Ice Cream Oracle: What Your Cone Says About Your Future

Silence Is Sovereignty: The Power of Being Unreadable

The Wind That Whispers Through Stone

Path of the Four Directions

Doctor Who: The Maestro's Symphony of Endings

Oxygen Grail: Breathing to Undo the Clock

Zodiacal Collapse: When Stars Devour Time

Teachings from the Red Sand Silence

Doctor Who: Omega – The Broken Equation

Memory Wipe Your Past: Start Over Like a MiB

Mitochondria Prime: Ignite the Core of Youth

A Nest of Roaches

Grub from the Galaxy: MiB Recipes You'll Never Forget

Whiskers of Power: Bastet's Guide to Inner Sovereignty

The Gift Must Cost Them: Negotiation Through Unequal Exchange

The Worm Guys' Wealth Code: Hustle Like an Alien

Bug Out: The Edgar Method for Ruthless Goal Setting

Weaving Life with Spiderwoman's Pattern

Doctor Who: The Rani's Renaissance

How to Get a Job (If You're a Puppygirl)

Speak Through Others: The Art of Proxy Power

T-Rex Your Trauma: Reclaim the Power of Your Primal Self

The Black Briefcase: How MiB Stay Wealthy in Silence

The Thirst Beyond Reason: Understanding Diabetes Insipidus From the Inside Out

Backwoods Witchcraft for Billionaires: The Pagan Path from Dirt Roads to Gold Roads

The Moonshine Grimoire: Fermented Spells for Abundance

The Nameless Geometry

The Wraith's Mixtape: Spellcasting with Songs of Sorrow

The Gallifreyan Gentleman: Silent Wealth, Sonic Confidence, and the Doctor's Code of Living

Sugar Water Confidence

Dino Totems: Spirit Guides from Earth's First Gods

Pumpkin Sigils & Ritual Smoke

The Hózhó Compass

The Distortus Discipline – Order from Inner Mutation

Witchcraft for the Cold-Blooded Soul

Moonlight Over the Blessingway

Water, Interrupted: When the Body Forgets How to Hold On

Deformed but Divine: Embracing Your Asymmetry

Hexes in the Henhouse: The Farm Witch's Guide to Power

The Reversed Flame: A Grimoire of Inverted Power

Salt, Cells, and Sanity: Reclaiming Balance with Diabetes Insipidus

King of the Broken: Crowning the Flawed Self

Moonlight Scars: Emo Moon Magick and the Art of Lunar Sorrow

Noose Spells: Magick of the Hanging Rope

The Goth Cathedral: Rituals of the Broken and Beautiful

The Cretaceous Codex: Dino Spirits and Fossil Magick

The Turkey Bones Ritual

Nine Lives of Manifestation: Unlocking Bastet's Reality Codes

Chaos Muscles: Building Strength from Twisted Pain

Emo Blood Magick: The Veins of Power

The 3AM Flood: Nighttime Urination, Sleep Loss, and the DI Spiral

The Silence Between the Stars

The Lemon Method: Sour Your Way to Success

Starlit Sovereign

The Rite of Twelve Gates: Walking the Gates of the Duat.

Cornbread and Conjure: Recipes for Riches and Rootwork

The Black Rose Rituals: Emo Love Spells and Obsession Magick

The Eternal Goodbye: Death Magick and Rebirth Rituals

Sinkrot: The Drain That Remembers

The Hybrid Mindset: Thinking Beyond Evolution

Bone Dry: Navigating Dehydration Before It Breaks You

Wreathcraft: Winter Sigils and Yuletide Spells

The Rite of Twelve Mouths

Get Some Tarot cards: https://www.makeplayingcards.com/sell/apophis-occult-shop

Get some shirts: https://www.bonfire.com/store/apophis-shirt-emporium/

Instagrams:
@apophis_enterprises,
@apophisbookemporium,
@apophisscardshop
Twitter: @apophisenterpr1
Tiktok:@apophisenterprise
Youtube: @sg1fan23477
Hive: @sg1fan23477
CheeLee: @SG1fan23477

Podcast: Apophis Chat Zone: https://open.spotify.com/show/5zXbrCLEV2xzCp8ybrfHsk?si=fb4d4fdbdce44dec

Newsletter: https://apophiss-newsletter-27c897.beehiiv.com/

If you want to support me or see posts of other projects that I have come over to: **buymeacoffee.com/mpetchinskg**
I post there daily several times a day

Get your Dinowicca or Christmas themed digital products, especially Santa Raptor songs and other musics. Here: **https://sg1fan23477.gumroad.com**

Apophis Yuletide Digital has not only digital Christmas items, but it will have all things with Dinowicca as well as other Digital products.